A Brief Guide to

TEEN
SUICIDE
PREVENTION

for Parents, Teachers, Clergy, and Friends

by Kathy Harris Henderson

ISBN: 978-1-936497-18-8

Searchlight Press
Who Are You Looking For?
5634 Ledgestone Drive
Dallas, Texas 75214-2026 USA
888-896-6081
www.Searchlight-Press.com

Manufactured in the United States of America

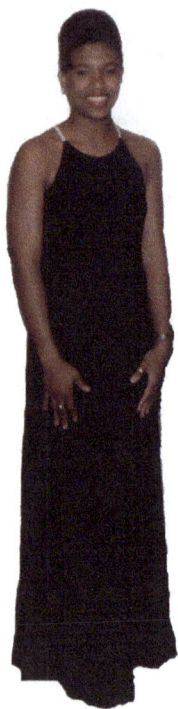

In Loving Memory
of Kourtney

FOREWORD

This book begins with a painful, personal experience of teen suicide. Building on real world experience, it then explores how the growth and development of a teenager and teens' experiences during adolescence affect their ability to make good choices. <u>A Brief Guide to Teen Suicide Prevention for Parents, Teachers, Clergy, and Friends</u> empowers the institutions of family, school, and faith community to support teens in a collaborative way.

TABLE OF CONTENTS

Charts-Graphs-Statistics

ACKNOWLEDGMENT

I will always be eternally grateful for the opportunity to further my education, especially since I am in the fall of life. God is truly faithful and He will give us the desires of our hearts as He gives us back the years the enemy tried to take. Our time is not His time, and He will complete the good work that He began in us. To God be the Glory!

I give thanks to God for my husband, Pastor Dr. David Henderson, Jr., for having a heart to want to make education attainable to those who desire to further their Christian Education. He saw the need to allow the Greater Mt. Pleasant Church to be a satellite school. This bold move brought the school to the lay persons, while making it economically affordable to those who truly wanted an education. So from the bottom of my heart I say thank you and I love you.

To my professors, Dr. J.B. Gassaway, Dr. Lloyd C. Blue, Dr. Craig White, Dr. John Cunyus, and Dr. Joseph Gill, for your tireless efforts of instruction are very much appreciated. I could sit and listen to you for hours. Thank you for heeding the call of God for your lives. More than anything I personally thank you for loving what you do so much that you just couldn't keep it to yourself. To Dr. Gassaway, I truly thank you for helping see how God has a plan for my pain, and to John (Dr. Cunyus), your response after reading my story, "I immediately put it in the 'must be published file,'" was exactly the confirmation I needed to walk through this door God had opened.

I am also extremely grateful for all those who supported me, encouraged me, and most of all prayed for me, especially my family. I shall always strive to bring clarity and understanding to God's Word when I stand to teach, and as I continue my journey in Christian Education.

And to my son, Cory you'll never know how your daily encouragement and belief meant to me. God is going to blow your mind when you see what He has in store for you.

Last, but not least this book is dedicated to the memory of my daughter, who gave me the privilege and pleasure of being her mother for sixteen years. My tears are less frequent, but nevertheless after fourteen years they still fall. Kourtney, you will forever be in my heart.

A Mother's Story

*The Unforeseen
and Unexpected*

It was the weekend of March 22, 1980; my son was having softball tryouts, and within another week my greatly anticipated, brand new baby girl was due. Kourtney Nicole arrived early the next morning at

> **I thought to myself what a miracle life is, as I studied her each day I asked, "How can anyone not believe there's a God?"**

2:13 a.m. She was not only beautiful, she was also perfect, and I thanked God for giving me what I requested, a girl. Daddy made it through the delivery and big brother anxiously awaited to see his new sister.

For eight weeks I got acquainted with my new package, as she kept exploring the new surroundings around her. I thought to myself what a miracle life is, as I studied her each day I asked, "How can anyone not believe there's a God?" I would look for hours without end at my new baby and wonder how bright her future would be.

The weeks swiftly went by, and before long my body was back at the bank working, but my mind longed to be home with Kourtney. Even though I wasn't at home with my baby, she was in the best of care with my mother, and I thanked God for making it possible.

I had always heard my parents, as well as my grandparents say, "children are soon grown and gone." Because I could remember how long I felt it took for me to reach the point of leaving home that just didn't seem to be a true statement. But so many things change when you have children of your own. The marriage was really rocky, and we argued constantly. It was only after the fact I realized how much damage parents do when they argue in their children's presence.

It seemed like I blinked and we were enrolling Kourtney in first grade. Little did I know that as Kourtney ended those first years of school, her father had plans to end his relationship with me. The end of first grade brought big changes. My little girl was excited about being in 'big school' and I was thrilled she was going to the second grade; on the other hand her father was preparing to leave and be part of another family. This was definitely not what I saw when I wondered about the future just a few years ago. I asked God the question He so often hears when life just happens, "Why Me?" I always had my mom and dad during my growing up years, and I wanted that so much for my children. It was soon that I realized that sometimes God allows things to happen in order to protect us.

> **I tried hard not to let her hear me speak about her father in a negative way.**

I worked in the public, and so did my husband as a minister and a policeman. I was determined not to allow anyone to tear my family apart, but it wasn't long before I realized that he was planning a big wedding ceremony. Painful as a divorce can be the atmosphere between us was not healthy for anyone in the family, so I said to myself, "it is what it is."

I was raised in a Christian home and always had belonged to a local church. It was difficult at first to think about returning to my former church, but I needed the support and the fellowship. Besides at least there was a former church to go home to.

Kourtney, being a daddy's girl, really took it hard those first few years. I tried hard not to let her hear me speak about her father in a negative way. My son became the protector of his mom and baby sister, while at the same time, struggling to become a young man. He was feeling a loss too. I felt such embarrassment. Since we lived in a small town, and both of us worked in such public places, I don't have to tell you how fast the news travelled.

By the grace of God we all managed to get through the tough years and boy were they tough. Not just because of the divorce, but now with only one income coming in every day was stressful and challenging. I didn't really know what affect the crises would have on us till later. Kourtney soon reached the age where going to her scheduled visits at her dad's were not a priority any more. She was soon to be thirteen, and with adolescence came new interests and priorities.

Soon to become a teenager and now in junior-high school, Kourtney was a very busy girl. She became a part of the school's political forum, preparing to take a class trip to Washington, D.C., and changed her sport of interest from softball to basketball. In spite of challenges my son had he made it through high school, and would soon be leaving for the Navy. Life was good again, or so it appeared to be.

Kourtney became a very good basketball player, kept up her good grades, her teachers spoke well of her, and she made a lot of new friends. I thanked God for allowing me to see smiles on her face again, and watch her enjoying life. She had finally arrived in high-school, every teenager's dream! Now there were even a few more privileges along with a little more independence, and freedom.

One of the things I noticed with Kourtney that first year was her choices in friends. I thought to myself, "well we had moved to a different area of town." She was doing well in school and they appeared to be good kids. Everyone was looking forward to freshman year being over and passing to the tenth grade.

> **No one could have imagined the changes that were to come in just a matter of months.**

Summer came and went and before long we were in another school year and preparing for yet another basketball season, except this time Kourtney felt that she would be moved up to varsity. She was really on cloud nine. To her, life was good, and to mom everything on the outside seemed to be just fine. Kourtney had arthroscopic surgery on her knee and varsity had to wait another year. She decided instead to become the person that would lead her class to win the "spirit stick" at the pep rallies each week. It wasn't long before she bounced back, with strength in her knee and she was her old self again.

Now a junior, Kourtney was looking forward to driving without mom in the car, later curfews, and sleepovers, all normal expectations for a sixteen year old, right? No one could have imagined the changes that were to come in just a matter of months.

It was a Friday morning while dropping Kourtney off at school that we discussed the fact that I would be out of town, and she was to stay at her grandmother's that night. I would be back early the next morning, which would be Saturday. Her dad would pick her up after school, and take her to my mother's. I told her that she could go out with her friends Saturday night, instead of Friday. We said our 'good-byes' and 'I love yous' and she was off.

While out of town at an annual banquet I received a phone call. It was the type of call that a parent never wants to receive. When I went to the phone my Pastor's voice was on the other end telling me to hurry home and go to the hospital because there had been an accident, he didn't say what type of accident. The whole ride home I was praying while my mind endeavored to consider what type of accident could have happened.

When I arrived at the hospital, one of my church members who worked at the hospital met me and brought me through the cafeteria in the back of the hospital and up to ICU. This route was taken because every floor of the hospital was filled with teenagers.

What I saw when I finally arrived in ICU was Kourtney, my beautiful, perfect little girl, lying in a bed, connected to a respirator, with the right side of her head swollen and bandaged from a self-inflicted gunshot wound. I stood there, praying and asking God that all too familiar question: "Why Me?" while at the same time praying to Him not to take her. The doctors were telling me she was brain dead, and I would probably need to make a decision to take her off the respirator. They said I could continue to wait, but if she got a chance and went home she would probably live in a vegetated state the rest of her life. I had to make a decision. I did not want to make a decision. I wanted God to deliver her.

Still at her side, the next morning there had not been any change. I was asked by the doctors if I had decided what I was going to do. They asked me if I knew Kourtney had put on her driver's license to be an organ donor, which I did not. The morning slipped away into the afternoon, and exactly at 1:28 p.m. Kourtney too had slipped away.

There were papers to sign concerning her being an organ donor, time was of the essence. Once that was taken care of it was not long before you could hear the sounds of the helicopter on the roof of the hospital taking my baby's vital organs to people desperately awaiting them.

Was this it? Does anyone care what I'm feeling? I watched out the window of the hospital until the helicopter was out of proximity of sight and sound. Then I asked God again "why didn't you take me?"

> **All the dreams of high-school and college graduations, along with planning a wedding with my daughter and the arrival of her first child were gone.**

Was this the invisible war I had heard preached about so many times? If it was, had I lost?

It might seem a bit morbid on the surface, but if you are a child of God, you have a final, secure, and unchanging hope that no circumstance, person, or tragedy can take from you. It doesn't matter if you're going bankrupt, or one of your children dies, your finances are in the ditch-whatever. From a human perspective, the worst that can happen to someone who is a believer is death, and the moment you die you're with Jesus, and that doesn't sound like losing.

All the dreams of high-school and college

graduations, along with planning a wedding with my daughter and the arrival of her first child were gone. There wouldn't be any of the dreams I once had planned sixteen years ago coming true, but those were my plans.

It's been a journey, and of course a lot of different emotions as well as questions still come. I think of so many things I could have done better, maybe even done differently, but only God knows if any of that would have changed anything. The tears are not on a daily basis anymore but they still fall. Now when I hold her picture I still can't believe such a tragedy happened to my daughter, but then I read the death certificate one more time, and I am brought back to reality.

I am glad to report I'm still holding on to my faith. It's still hard to talk about her without tears forming in my eyes, but God gave me tear ducts for times such as these. I ask Him to give me the courage to share my wisdom with anyone that will listen, not that I'm an expert, but there may be something I can say to help or even encourage a parent or a teen. In spite of it all God is still good.

CHAPTER ONE

*Parental
Responsibilities
and Needs
in the Home*

The growth and development of children is significant at any age, but the teenage years tend to be a little more complex. Developing interpersonal relationships with their parents is a vital part of a teenager's life. When two people have strong needs and each fills the other's needs, a powerful interpersonal relationship is formed. When the needs are weak from both persons, and each fills those needs, the relationship is mild. When both people have strong needs and they are not being filled the result is a poor relationship. In essence the key to having good interpersonal relationships is simply to understand the role that needs play.

> **The growth and development of children is significant at any age, but the teenage years tend to be a little more complex.**

The parent must both understand their role while also making their role be understood by all concerned. The primary role of the parent is to provide basic needs for their child. Needs are defined as demands of the body for physical and psychological well-being. We can categorize them into four groups.

In some cases, if some needs are not met, the person may die. For instance people must have water and food to live. On the other hand, the satisfaction of other needs can make a person's life rich and fulfilling. The four categories of a child's needs are:

1. Physical Needs for Survival

* People need air, water, food, sleep, shelter, clothing, and safety.
* Children need fresh air, clean water, nutritious food, sufficient sleep, and a safe environment.

2. Social Needs for Mental Health

* People need to be loved, to love, to feel a part of and to include others.
* Children need to be loved by their parents, they need to interact with others, and they need to show their love to others.

3. Curiosity

* People want to know what they do not know.
* Parents should encourage their children to explore and to act in an age appropriate manner.

4. Self-Awareness

* Everybody needs healthy self-esteem, self-fulfillment and positive recognition to

realize their existence and value.

* Parents need to help their child develop a sense of self as a person of value and competency. They should encourage their child to learn and praise their right behavior, abilities and accomplishments.

Most parents will agree that the teenage years are a developmental phase fraught with challenges; yet beyond the traditional challenges of this adolescent phase today's teenagers face unique demands and difficulties as never before.

In order to help teenagers develop physically, mentally, and socially parents should not only meet the basic needs mentioned, they must also respond to their teen's unique needs. Though parents often regard the teenage years as a carefree time when compared with the period of childhood, parents can look back on their own adolescent years and recall how tumultuous and uncertain they can be. This may help parents be prepared to react to their teenager with support and understanding.

Everyone wants and needs to be understood, especially teenagers. A parent should always want their teenager to be totally honest with them, and never use the information against the teen in any way.

When this is done the dynamics of the parent – teen relationship will change.

NOTES

CHAPTER TWO

*Teen's Needs
and Responsibilities
in the Home*

It is important to consider the needs of the teenager as well as those of each person with whom the teenager is in relationship. Each person's needs in the relationship should be met.

> **Teenagers need to be able to test the values passed to them by their parents and taught in schools.**

1. Test Values

> * Teenagers need to be able to test the values passed to them by their parents and taught in schools. They will often engage in various experiments and seek out new experiences, for example: new clothes, hair styles, friends, and activities.
>
> * Even though most teenagers will ultimately decide values for themselves, their parents and schools will have an impact on them.

2. Seek Out Identity – Who Am I?

> * While teenagers are striving to leave childhood behind, they will start to seek out their identity. Now, more than ever they need their parents to understand that this sometimes confusing behavior is a result of their need to develop their own identity. It is the responsibility of the teen to obey the

guidelines that have been set by their parents

3. Acceptance

* Acceptance or recognition is a basic need for everyone; this is especially true for teenagers. For example, whatever their opinion is, a parent should be willing to listen to their teen even if and or when they don't agree with him or her. Teenagers really would like for their parents to try to think the way they are thinking, and not judge them right away. Teenagers would like to be provided encouragement instead of criticism, which not only builds their self-esteem, it also helps to motivate. After the parent has listened to the teen and decides differently, the teen's responsibility is to respect and comply with the parent's final decision.

4. Give and Receive Affection

* Teenagers have a need to give affection as well as receive it. Helping them cope with their emotions is very important. They need to be assured that everyone has feelings such as disappointment, sadness, anger, joy, and excitement, and that expressing them appropriately to others is the key.

* Teenagers need to be shown unconditional

love whatever the situation: even if they have disappointed, disrespected or even angered their parents. This unconditional love is vital because teenagers need their parents affection and to feel secure. If they have failed in school, they need encouragement from their parents instead of lecturing. Remember a child is never too old to need a loving, nurturing family. One on one time with the teen, letting them hear you brag on them, and surprise notes or treats are examples of things that can be done to show care for the teenager.

5. Want and Need Independence

* Teenagers struggle to figure out where they are in life, and who they are. They are thinking about their future and trying to find answers. In other words they are trying to be independent. In this critical time, they do not want their parents to treat or educate them the same way they do their younger siblings. Even though the teenager is older, the bottom line is to understand they are the child and the parent is the parent and each has different needs, roles, and responsibilities

6. Need Guidance and Limits

* Teenagers need parents to provide limits,

because they sometimes won't make the best decisions. Too much freedom causes insecurity. Although teenagers think they can take care of themselves, they really need a loving family, as well as a lot of guidance to steer them onto a better life plan. Being conscience of these needs will help the teenager succeed. On the other hand if limits are exceeded or boundaries are crossed, the teenager should understand they will have to face the consequences.

NOTES

CHAPTER THREE

*Responsibilities
of the School
and Teen*

Schools have an important place in the community; they really can be viewed as a smaller community within the larger community working to produce productive citizens.

> **What has been allowed at home with parents or school with other adults will have a significant effect on the teenager.**

Educational institutions should always have the student's best interests at heart. By the time a child completes the teenage development stage they have learned quite a bit from their home life as well as their school life. What has been allowed at home with parents or school with other adults will have a significant effect on the teenager. It is important that those in authority recognize this in order to better understand the teen. Even with this in mind, there are some basic needs and responsibilities that an educational institution has toward the teen.

1. **To Educate.**

Educational institutions' main responsibility is to educate the teen so they can be prepared to attend a university, college, or technical school. The goal is for the teen to not only be able to further their education, but also to have an opportunity for a career, and be a productive member of society.

2. **Provide Safety.**

Schools must provide an environment that is safe and free of anything which could harm the child. This includes external or internal factors. For example external factors could be ex-students that are labeled drop-outs who linger around the schools only for negative reasons. Internal factors could be a situation where bullying is happening. In any case the school is responsible to effectively address the problem while keeping the teen safe.

3. **Provide Accurate Records.**

Maintaining accurate attendance records and documenting communication with the teen and parents concerning the student's attendance, allows all concerned to narrow the window of opportunity for any negative behavior on the teen's part.

4. **Reporting Signs of Abuse.**

Schools must actively and intentionally work to be aware of any signs of abuse or violence to the child and report it to the necessary authorities; even at the risk of reporting the parent or guardian, or school employees.

5. **On a Personal Note.**

The school as well as the parent should always be on the lookout for any changes in a teen's demeanor, no matter how small. This could be a change in their attitude, dress, hair, or personal hygiene, which could be a sign of depression. I think both parties would agree that it is better to be safe than sorry in any situation. When the parent has done an effective job in training their teen to be responsible at home; the teen is empowered to easily and effectively transition into the environment of the school.

A large part of this parental training is establishing rules for their teens. Believe it or not our teenagers need rules to live by, a structured environment, and to be held accountable for their actions. When these rules are enforced they put in place an environment where the teen understands that there are consequences for their actions.

In summary, the teen's responsibility in school is simple; to go to school regularly, follow all rules and regulations, complete all homework and assignments, and be respectful to all teachers as well as fellow students. If these rules are not complied with, the consequences already established should be enforced.

I strongly believe that during this complex and sometimes difficult phase of development in a child's life, it is very important for the school and parent to join   forces and work together for the teen, focusing not just on schoolwork, but on the whole person. Joining the resources of the school and home; utilizing clear and open communication would help to strengthen the probability for lessening the chances of the teen falling into pitfalls that sometimes occur in adolescence. This partnership would help, especially where depression is an issue, to produce a more favorable outcome for all concerned.

NOTES

CHAPTER FOUR

*Responsibilities
of the Faith Community*

> **Teenagers need to be prepared spiritually, morally, socially, psychologically, and emotionally for the world in which they live.**

The Need
for a Youth Minister

The increasing difficulty of keeping youth interested in and actively participating in the church has intensified the need for a more effective ministry with youth. Increasingly our youth are either misused or lost. They are challenged by things which are great and things we might find insignificant. Youth activities demand much time and considerable energy on the part of those who work with them. Many churches have been convinced of the need to secure a youth minister to develop and guide a progressive youth program.

Teenagers need to be prepared spiritually, morally, socially, psychologically, and emotionally for the world in which they live. Because the teen is at the peak of their intellectual vigor, they have to cope with decisions concerning their choices in life. It is at this time that there is a critical need for someone to supervise the youth activities.

1. Must be a Christian.

It goes without saying that if you are planning to be a youth leader working with Christian or even non-Christian teens, you should be a Christian yourself. This doesn't mean that you must be the most knowledgeable Christian in the world, but you do need to have some understanding of your faith, and a heart centered on God.

When dealing with teenagers, an effective youth leader should be able to demonstrate their own relationship with God as an example to teens. It's hard to teach someone something you don't practice yourself. The philosophy, "Do as I say, not as I do", doesn't go very far with teenagers in this day and time.

2. Have a Servant's Heart.

Someone working with teens should have a "servant's heart". Youth ministry takes a lot of work, and usually involves anything from clean-up to attending events beyond regular services.

Without a servant's heart you are not setting a Christian example to the students. Being a servant is a huge part of being a Christian. Christ was a servant to man and He called people to be servants to one another. It doesn't mean you have to be a slave to ministry, but you must come ready to help out whenever possible.

3. **Be Responsible.**

In many cases youth ministers are not much older than the teenage group. The youth minister must understand that as the leader, they must be responsible. Those working with youth have responsibility for certain tasks and supervision, and must be authoritative enough to keep the teens in line. Just because a teen is a Christian does not mean they make the best decisions.

Just like the parent, and the school teacher, youth leaders also need to set boundaries that show there is a line between student and teacher. Those working with teens in the church may at times see the need to notify parents, or even stand up to the teen when they are doing wrong.

4. **Have a Positive Attitude.**

Few things are more damaging to a youth ministry than a cranky leader. If the youth leaders complain the entire time, the teens will start to associate negative traits with the youth group and the church as a whole. Even in the worst of times it is essential that the youth leader be able to put on a calm face and keep their focus on the good in every situation. Yes, this can be hard, but with teenagers. youth leaders need to keep the students focused and headed in the right direction.

> **So many times teenagers feel that they are never heard.**

5. **Be a Good Listener.**

So many times teenagers feel that they are never heard. As a youth minister, there may be times that call for personal counseling. Sometimes this is an inescapable responsibility. Since they are respected by young people as their leader, many youth will naturally come to the youth minister or youth leader for guidance and advice. There may be times the youth minister cannot refer these young people to the pastor because the youth may interpret such a move as rejection.

Given this reality, the youth minister should have a basic knowledge and understanding of the principles of counseling. While all the problems that young people have cannot be anticipated; there are basic areas that cause concern for young people.

> (a) **Personal Attitudes:** As a young person reaches adolescence, their physical growth and maturity sometimes leads to new mental outlooks which may tend to confuse and

perplex them. Because of these factors they are developing a new self-concept. They no longer think of themselves as a child, but neither can they consider themselves as an adult. Their attitudes and concepts about themselves are very important because they will affect all of their relationships.

(b) **Social relationships:** Young people are very concerned about social relationships, especially with peers. In the early teens, boys and girls have to learn to relate to members of the opposite sex in a new way. Also, they desire acceptance by their peer groups, often leading to seeking conformity at any cost. Parental relationships usually will be difficult during this period. In view of this, the youth minister may have opportunities to counsel with both parents as well as youth.

(c) **Religious Convictions:** Young people are beginning to examine religious beliefs and convictions that they have previously accepted without question. This is healthy, and might lead to deeper and more realistic beliefs. The young person is also trying to face the complex problem of trying to apply their beliefs and convictions to their actions.

This area is the particular responsibility of the church. The young person may receive counseling at school or from other professional counselors, but the church has an obligation to guide youth in the area of religious matters.

In all areas of counseling, the approach should guide the youth to find a solution to their own problems. There may be instances when the youth minister will need to refer individuals for professional help, when this happens they must not hesitate to do so. The area of personal counseling affords one of the greatest opportunities for a youth minister to lead a young person into a relationship with God. Through a personal relationship established in a counseling situation, the youth minister can share his or her faith, and in some cases reach the child where the parent cannot.

Responsibilities of the Church Family

Every church regardless of size is involved to some degree in a youth program and should make financial provisions for it in the church budget. Some young people are tithers. Therefore, the inclusion in the church budget of an item for the youth program is not merely a matter of good business for the church; it is an educational experience for the young people. The

> **Nothing else causes more trouble in leadership than unclear expectations.**

youth learn early that tithing is necessary for ministry to go forth, and that the church includes them in the ministry. Educating the youth in the church is such an important role; that support should be given to the ministry by the church at all times.

1. Value Youth Leaders.

Because there is a lot of responsibility when a person becomes a youth leader, the church as a whole should let the leaders know how much they are valued. Verbally let them know how much they are appreciated for the work they do. They are responsible for strengthening the teens in the congregation and in their Christian walk.

2. Have Clear Expectations.

Nothing else causes more trouble in leadership than unclear expectations. Therefore it is important that the church leadership provide clear expectations for its youth leaders. The clearer the expectations; the easier   it is for people to fulfill them. The more a person knows about what he or she is supposed to do, the more responsible they will be.

3. **Be Flexible.**

Not all youth workers are perfect, so the church leadership should be flexible in their expectations. Far too often one or two youth workers end up doing all the work. In this case the church should make sure they have conversations with those that are neglecting their responsibilities, so as not to make it a habit.

4. **Be Open-Minded.**

While small actions on the church's part make a youth leader feel valued, there is nothing like listening and keeping an open mind about the ministry. If your youth leadership has ideas, consider trying them as you keep the youth group's best interest at heart. Youth leaders often feel more responsible when they feel they are contributing to the overall mission of the church. The goal should be for the teens to be loyal to the church. Research has shown that two thirds of the teens who stay in church as young adults describe the church as a vital part of their relationship with God.

The Parents' Responsibility

Christian parents are appointed as guardians to watch and **foster the growth of the teen's faith**. It is through a parent's faith that the Holy Spirit loves to take possession of the child's faith. As the child grows, his faith will grow. God connects all believing, knowing, and loving with doing. Obedience is God's test of righteousness and reality. Therefore the parent should teach their teen God's standard of conduct, and the best way to do this is **by following God's standard of conduct themselves**.

Example is better than precept. In our ordinary Christianity, children are taught to believe that God's commandments are unpleasant. Parents should **make sure that the Bible is not just a rule book to be held over the teen's head**, keeping them from everything they like and demanding from them everything that is difficult. Rules and regulations presented without love always brings about sin and bitterness.

> **Many Christians are so busy making money that they have no time to speak about soul concerns with their children.**

Many Christians are so busy making money that they have no time to speak about soul concerns with their children. If their children died without hope, how would the parents quiet their conscience? Christian parents are under double responsibility, not only because they are their children, but also because God has given the parents salvation. Since the parent has been given the light they are bound to give the light to all around, with the first priority to be to those they have birthed into the world.

It is of utmost importance for the parent to speak personally to them about their salvation, and once is not enough. It must be repeated until the right chord is touched in the child's heart, persevering in affectionate admonitions unto every child in the household. This is not to say that Christian parents are perfect, but they are obligated to do their part, and not leave the responsibility to anyone else.

Parental care can alone preserve household piety, and if that be gone, the pillars of the nation are removed. On the other hand there are those parents who are not Christians. These parents neglect altogether the religious education of their children. So many feel that when they have sent their children to Sunday School they have done all that needs to be done for them, and even if this is neglected they seem to be content. There are other parents who have never prayed for their children, perhaps because so many times they don't yet know what it is to pray for themselves in sincerity and truth. When parents conform to the world, usually their children will follow suit. When the parents see their faults being repeated in their children, it is then that the parents realize that more training should have been done

CHAPTER FIVE

*The Teen's Will
and Conscience*

We must consider what part the teen's will and conscience play in their decision making abilities. The following is an excerpt taken from the book, How to Bring Your Children to Christ by Andrew Murray, pertaining to the will and conscience of a child.

> *The parent has been entrusted with the solemn task of teaching their teen how to use his or her will in the right way. This delicate instrument is put into the hands of the parents to keep, to direct, and to strengthen. The parent must train the child to exercise his will in the right way. God has taught more than once in His Word that obedience is the child's first virtue. He is to obey not because he understands or approves, but because the parent commands. In this he is to become the master of his own will by voluntary submitting it to a higher authority. The goal is for the child to obey, and obedience from this principle will secure a double blessing for the child. While guiding the will to form right habits, it strengthens the control the child has over his will. When this has been attained, a sure foundation has been laid for the exercise of the child's free will choosing what appears to him to be best.*

> **The development of the will depends upon the impulses and motives which prompt it to action.**

In the first stage of childhood, before the child knows to refuse evil and choose good, simple obedience is law. As the child matures into the teenage years it is still a parent's influence that must train the will to exercise the power which everything in life later depends. The child must now be trained himself to refuse evil and choose good.

The development of the will depends upon the impulses and motives which prompt it to action. These impulses and motives will depend upon the objects presented to the mind, and the degree of attention they are given. The scripture instructs us that in our fallen nature the soul is stimulated far more by the visible and the temporal, than by the unseen and the real, and the soul is deceived by what is beautiful. This is why the teen should be trained early in life. Teens don't realize that the influence of what is present outweighs that of the future, even though it may be of greater worth.

It is the work of the parent to present to their teen the best reasons for taking certain actions and help them to refuse evil and choose good. The parent must present to the child the beauty of virtue, the nobility and happiness of self-denial, the pleasure that duty brings, and the fear and favor of God. Creating positive emotions within the teen will cause them to gladly will themselves to choose that which is good.

When dealing with the teen's conscience, the parent must act as the conscience for the child, calling them to be true to their higher instincts and convictions. The training of the teen aims especially at teaching them to refuse evil and choose good when there is no parent nearby to help. The conscience of every person is a guardian and helper of inestimable value in choosing the path of right. Wise training can do much to establish the authority of this inner rule. Proper training will lead the teen to look upon his conscience, not as a spy, but as his truest friend and best companion. The goal is for the authority of the parent and the conscience to be linked together, so that even in the parent's absence, the weight of his influence may be felt. Therefore the aim and success of moral training must be to form in the child the habit of self-rule and encouraging them to always wait and listen for the gentle inner whisper that tells them to refuse evil and choose the good.

By the parent knowing the meaning of the words good

and evil, he will see how in every step of life two motives are struggling to be master. Choosing between evil and good are lifelong tasks which are carried out every day. The parent must recognize the great responsibility entrusted to them to strengthen the young and developing will of their child. If the parent does this well, they will have done a great work having laid a strong foundation to promote good development of the teen's decision making abilities. Parents must keep in mind their highest work is to take charge of their child's will.

NOTES

CHAPTER SIX

*Development
of the Teen's Brain*

When considering the decision making abilities of teenagers it is important to know that the adolescent brain is not fully developed until after the age of eighteen. In an article found in *Family Education Newsletter*, Barbara Cooke presents recently discovered research that adults think with their prefrontal cortex, which is the rational part of the brain, while teenagers process their information with the *amygdale*, the instinctual, emotional part of the brain. The *amygdale*, located in the back of the brain, primarily controls how a teen acts during their middle school and high school years.

When considering the decision making abilities of teenagers it is important to know that the adolescent brain is not fully developed until after the age of eighteen.

Adolescent brain development does not happen in all parts of the brain at the same time. The maturation of connection proceeds from the back of the brain to the front of the brain. Thus the last area of the brain to develop is the frontal lobe, which is the large area responsible for modulating reward, planning, impulsiveness, attention, acceptable social behavior, and other roles that are known as execution decisions.

How many times has a parent, or teacher, or even an authority figure at church asked a teenager, "What in the world were you thinking?" Nine times out of ten, teens are not thinking, not like adults anyway, because they absolutely, positively cannot do that yet. Their brains are not hard wired like adults.

It is partially because of this developmental timeline that a teenager can be quick to conjure up a stinging remark, or a biting insult, and be so uninhibited in firing it off at the nearest target whether a friend, former friend, or a bewildered parent.

The impulse to hurt or insult is there, just as it may be for an adult in a stressful situation, but the brain regions that an adult might rely on to stop himself, haven't caught up in a teenager.

The following is an excerpt from an interview with Dr. Jay Gield, practicing child and adolescent psychiatrist and chief brain imaging specialist in the Child Psychiatry Division of the National Institute of Mental Health.

> *The most surprising thing is how much the teen's brain changes. By age six the brain is almost 90% of its adult size. But the gray matter, or thinking part of the brain, continues to thicken throughout childhood as*

> **The Use It or Lose It Principle: Those cells and connections used will survive and flourish. Those that are not used will wither and die.**

the brain cells get extra connections, much like a tree growing extra branches, twigs or roots.

Since the frontal part of the brain is the last area to fully develop, skills such as forethought and caution are still developing. These very skills are the skills that teens get better and better over time by doing. The process of thickening of the gray matter peaks at about age 11 in girls and 12 in boys, roughly about the same time as puberty. After that peak, the gray matter thins as the excess connections are eliminated or pruned.

But the pruning phase is perhaps even more interesting, because it has become known as the "use or it lose it principle". Those cells and connections used will survive and flourish. Those that are not used will wither and die. So if a teen is participating in music or sports or academics, those are the cells and connections that will be hard wired. Right around the time of puberty and on into the adult years is a particularly critical time for the brain sculpting to take place. For these reasons it is unfair for adults to expect teens to have adult levels of organizational or decision-making skills before their brains are finished being built.

Because the frontal lobe is like the CEO, or the executive of the brain, it is involved in things such as planning, strategizing and organizing, along with initiating and shifting attention and with stopping and starting. In calm situations teenagers can rationalize almost as well as adults. But stress can hijack what is called a "hot cognition" and decision making. The frontal lobes will help put the brakes on a desire for thrills and taking risks which tend to be the building block of adolescence. Educating teens concerning the developing stages of their brains might motivate them to change their own priorities. How a teenager utilizes their brain during this time can have many good and bad implications for the rest of their life

NOTES

CHAPTER SEVEN

Teen Suicide

> **Research shows that over ninety percent of people who kill themselves have depression.**

The decision making abilities of teenagers sometimes can be impulsive as well as irreversible. One such irreversible decision is the decision to commit suicide. Suicide behavior is complex. Research shows that over ninety percent of people that kill themselves have depression. Suicide is a major public health problem. Each year more than 30,000 Americans take their own lives. Among adolescents, suicide ranks as the third leading cause of death, behind unintentional injury, and homicide.

When a teenager commits suicide everyone is affected. Family members, friends, teammates, neighbors, and sometimes even those who didn't know the teen well might experience feelings of grief, confusion, guilt and a sense that if only they had done something differently the suicide could have been prevented.

The risk of suicide increases dramatically when children and teenagers have access to firearms at home, for nearly sixty percent of all suicides in the United States are committed with a gun. This alarming statistic calls for very careful measures to be taken with firearms. Any and all guns in the home should be kept unloaded, locked, and out of reach of children and teenagers. Ammunition should be stored separately from any guns and kept under lock and key. The keys for both the ammunition and gun(s) should be kept in different areas from household keys; and the keys to any firearms must be kept out of the reach of children and teens.

It should be noted that a teenager with an adequate support network of friends, family, religious affiliations, peer groups, and/or extracurricular activities may have an outlet to deal with everyday frustrations. However the sad reality is that many teens don't believe they have a support group; leaving them feeling disconnected and isolated from family and friends.

**These are the teens
that are at a high risk
to commit suicide!**

	United States		
	Suicide Rates, By Age Group: 1981-2005		
	(Suicides per 100,000 in age group per year)		
YEAR	10-14 Year-Olds	15-19 Year-Olds	20-24 Year-Olds
1981	0.89	8.62	15.65
1982	1.09	8.67	15.2
1983	1.09	8.65	14.64
1984	1.29	8.94	15.49
1985	1.62	9.87	15.39
1986	1.52	10.08	15.54
1987	1.53	10.17	14.97
1988	1.44	11.13	14.6
1989	1.41	11.08	14.86
1990	1.5	11.14	15.1
1991	1.49	11	14.83
1992	1.67	10.71	14.83
1993	1.68	10.78	15.61
1994	1.67	10.9	16.12
1995	1.72	10.29	15.81
1996	1.53	9.6	14.21
1997	1.55	9.29	13.31
1998	1.6	8.76	13.2
1999	1.2	8.04	12.3
2000	1.46	8.02	12.51
2001	1.3	7.95	11.93
2002	1.23	7.44	12.28
2003	1.15	7.26	12.07
2004	1.34	8.2	12.48
2005	1.29	7.66	12.35

a) Despite declines among all age groups nationwide, for adolescents between the ages of 15 and 19 the suicide rate has increased by six percent, and among children between the ages of ten and fourteen, the rate has increased by more than one hundred percent. So many times the question is asked, "How often do young people actually take their own lives?" The chart on page 64 provides the most recent data for three age groups for the period from 1981 to 2005.

This time frame is of particular interest to me, because it includes the year 1997, the year my daughter committed suicide.

The following data on page 66 is taken from "cause of death" information recorded by physicians on death certificates. Given that many persons committing suicide do not leave a suicide note, and some choose means of death that could be considered accidental, these data are likely to underestimate the actual number of suicides. The data is presented in rates that measure deaths due to suicide per 100,000 people in a particular category.

Suicide among teenagers often occurs following a stressful life event; such as a perceived failure at school, a breakup with a boyfriend or girlfriend, the death of a loved one, a divorce, or a major family conflict.

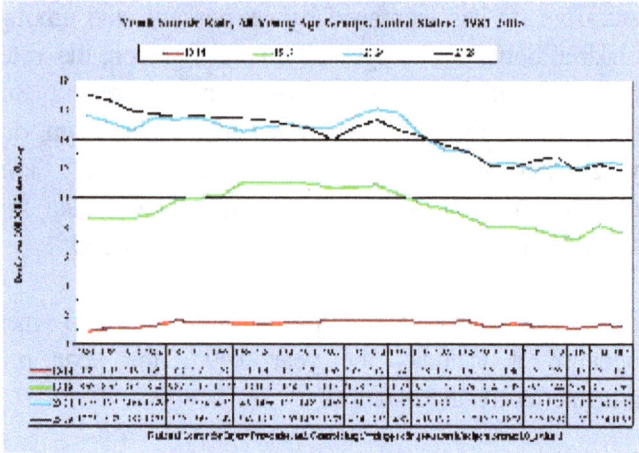

While teenagers are known for their hormonal changes and mood swings, it is important to watch for prolonged negative moods, because those may be warning signs of suicidal thoughts or potential suicide. Depression is most often the first warning sign of a potentially suicidal teen.

While it is scary to think that teenagers may be exhibiting warning signs for suicide; it is even more frightening to think that teens may decide to commit suicide on an impulse. These "in the moment" suicides generally occur when the teenager is in a situation where they are desperately upset. Unfortunately the only warning sign of unplanned suicides is depression.

Being able to recognize when a teen is depressed is very important because often times it may lead teenagers to focus on their failures and disappointments and to downplay their own worth. Depression causes teenagers to sink into a mindset that everything is hopeless and there is no reason to fix their lives. They usually can't see past the "right now".

Ten out of 100,000 teenagers decide to kill themselves. These numbers cannot be ignored. Educating our teens in school and in the home can help reduce these numbers; while allowing teens to express their feelings, and communicate their problems freely with someone, can help save their lives as well.

Whatever the reason may be that a teen decides to take their life is never an acceptable one. Many teen suicides might have been prevented if the lines of communication would have been open between them and someone who cared about them. Given this reality, if you suspect a teen is contemplating suicide you must treat their feelings of desperation with the utmost respect.

If for any reason you sense that a teen is contemplating suicide, get help immediately. In an emergency you can call 1-800-SUICIDE.

This chart shows the topics teenagers generally discuss when they call the suicide hotline. This confirms that not only parents, but also schools, as well as the church should be aware of teenagers with suicidal tendencies.

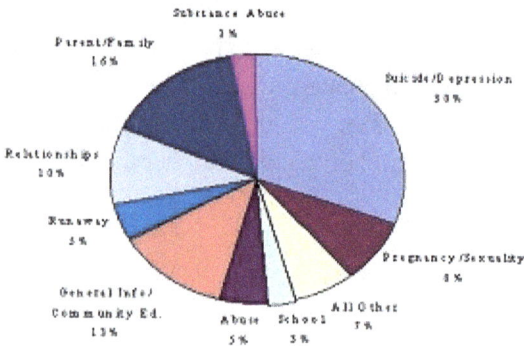

We all feel overwhelmed by difficult emotions or situations. But most people get through it or can put their problems in perspective and find a way to carry on with determination and hope.

So why does one person try suicide when another person in the same tough situation does not? What makes some teens more resilient than others? What makes one teenager unable to see another way out of a bad situation and thus consider ending their life? The chart on page 66 provides answers to these questions, revealing that to a large extent **most teenagers who attempt suicide are suffering with depression.**

Suicide rates differ between boys and girls. Girls think about and attempt suicide nearly twice as often as boys. Their tendency is to attempt suicide by overdosing drugs, or cutting themselves. However boys die by suicide almost four times as often as girls. Perhaps this is because their tendency is to use more lethal methods, such as fire arms, hanging, or jumping from heights.

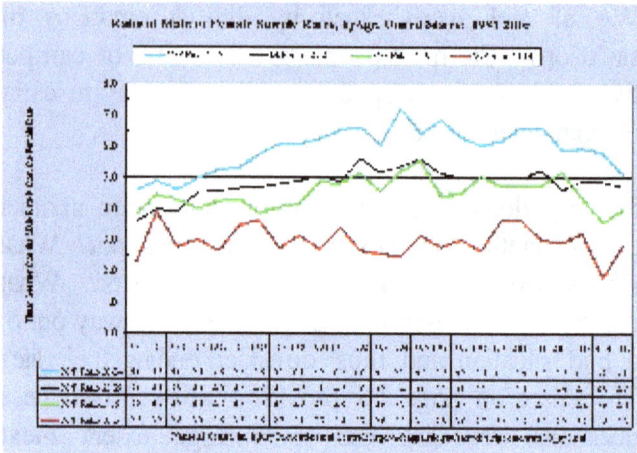

It might be hard for most of us to remember what it was like to be a teenager, being caught in that gray area between childhood and being an adult. While it is surely a time of tremendous possibility, it can also be a period of great confusion and anxiety; both of which would affect a teenager's decision-making ability.

CHAPTER EIGHT

*What I
Have Learned*

What I learned from my hurt was, don't ask why; ask what. When hurts hit a family hard, the most natural question to ask is, why? Stories in the Bible illustrate this over and over, but none illustrate it more painstakingly than the book of Job. God is patient with Job until he starts asking why.

> **I have learned not to ask God why did this or that happen, but to ask what direction do you want me to go, now that this has happened.**

Then God issues a stern reminder that His motive and character were not to be questioned. The right questions are not if we can understand all God's ways and reasons, but if we will trust Him and obey Him no matter what. My pastor husband once said, "from time to time back room conversations go on between God and Satan concerning believers". With this in mind, the big question posed by the book of Job is not, "why does a man suffer? The big question in the book of Job is why does a man serve God?"

I have learned not to ask God why did this or that happen, but to ask what direction do you want me to go, now that this has happened. When I decide to ask the "what" question instead of the "why" question, I don't see life's troubles as God's clenched fist of wrath but rather His open hand of opportunity and guidance. Then I see that even the hurtful experiences of life can draw us closer to God for guidance and character development and closer to others for support and strength.

I have also learned there is no need to be angry with God, because it won't change a thing. You see I must admit I was angry at God for allowing this to happen. I never will forget the first time I went to church after my daughter's death. The floor was opened for testimony service, and in the course of me speaking I stated, "I'm angry with God", and those seated near me began to part like the Red Sea. Since then I've grown spiritually, and I realize that when we try and shake an angry fist at God it will only deepen our hurt and increase our frustrations. Now I look for God's purposes in the painful situations of life; in doing so I find that my faith is stretched, and my character matures to increasingly imitate Christ.

Through this research I learned that Kourtney's brain wasn't fully developed, especially the part responsible for making rational decisions. I believe with all my heart she wanted a right now solution to her problem and at the time this would give it to her. I also learned that I should have talked more, even when she didn't want to, because maybe I could have said something that would have made a difference in the final

> **I learned that if and/or when a person should begin to make drastic changes, we must be careful not to rationalize them away.**

outcome. It's hard but I have stopped blaming myself, because I realize that the final decision was hers. I just don't feel it was a decision that she would have made if she was a little older, or even if I would have been there. All the questions that I might still think of in the future won't change anything, but it is comforting to know that God still invites me to come to Him with my questions, even after fourteen years.

I learned that if and/or when a person should begin to make drastic changes, we must be careful not to rationalize them away. When Kourtney began to change the friends she had grown up with, I should have taken a closer look. Because of the differences in the school structure when I attended school, I didn't have to contend with the same issues. All adults looked out   for all children and teenagers. In my adolescence not only were you expected to show and give respect to your parents and all adults; as teenagers we gladly did so.   As teenagers we experienced openness with our parents and a willingness to please them and the community.

Looking back I understand that the new friends Kourtney had were really a negative peer group. They came from good homes, with parents who were well respected in the community, however in many cases there was a lack of accountability and respect required from their teens.

I learned sometimes that when a dream dies, to just start dreaming another dream. When we have dreams that didn't work out the way we had planned it doesn't mean that God doesn't have another plan. I've learned you can't allow one disappointment or even a series of disappointments to put you in a state of hopelessness, because as long as you have God, you have hope.

I've learned that whenever I stand to give instructions to parents or children, to not listen to the devil, but to stand bold and speak loud. Because I know firsthand that what I have to say may save a life. It is a sad reality and an unfortunate fact that in our community and especially in the Black church, many people feel that persons who attempt or commit suicide are 'weak' or they are not strong in their faith. It is very important that we begin to learn the many factors that contribute to suicide especially in regard to our children and teenagers. The rates of suicide in our community are increasing by alarming numbers. Anything that I can say or do to keep another parent from enduring the pain I have endured, I will do.

> **Listening to a teen is a parent's primary source of feedback about how they're doing, what they're doing, and most importantly, who they're doing it with.**

God has blessed me with grandchildren, and I make it a point to listen to them, and dream with them. Listening to a teen is a parent's primary source of feedback about how they're doing, what they're doing, and most importantly, who they're doing it with. Don't be surprised that you don't anticipate everything they feel. This is increasingly true as children get older, and are more aware of the dynamics of interpersonal relationships. The signs are usually there when a teen is really reaching out for help and wanting someone to see their pain and hurt. If there is nothing wrong, there's no harm done, but if there is something wrong I am so glad I took the time to help.

When parents are young other things seem to take priority so I try to always have time for them. I don't have a problem being vocal about my concerns, whether to the children or adults because I have learned that all the adults in a teenager's life have to be on the same team no matter what the family situation.

One thing is for sure, God is God, and it is His will that we all have life. We are the only creations that are able to make choices, and while He would rather we didn't make some of the choices that we do, we are given that right. Sovereignty is a truth that is most effective in helping me through hurtful times. Now more than ever I stand on the foundational truth that God's knowledge, power, presence, and love are unquestionable and inexhaustible. In God's sovereignty we can all find the security and confidence we need to endure pain and even grow stronger through it, because truly God does work things out for the good of all those who love Him.

I have discovered that one of the most comforting sentences I can offer to others during times of great pain or loss is simply this: God is not surprised by this, and it is not outside His control. No matter what pain they might be facing I have been able to watch these words bring visible relief and security to their faces.

BIBLIOGRAPHY

Adams, Nate. <u>The Home Team: Practices for a Winning Family</u>. Grand Rapids, Michigan: Baker Publishing Company, 1996.

Carson, R. Logan. <u>The Christian Family in These Last Days</u>. Lithonia, Georgia: Orman Press, 2003.

Fitzpatrick, Elyse and Jim Newheiser. <u>When Good Kids Make Bad Choices</u>. Eugene, Oregon: Harvest House Publishers, 2005.

Ingram, Chip. <u>The Invisible Warfare</u>. Grand Rapids, Michigan: Baker Publishing Company, 2006.

Mahoney, Kelly. "Fostering Responsible Youth Leaders, How to Make Sure Your Leadership is Reliable". About.com.

Murray, Andrew. <u>How to Bring Your Children to Christ</u>. New Kensington, Pennsylvania: Whitaker House, 1984.

"Teen Suicide Prevention" State Health Lawmakers Digest, Fall 2005: Vol 5 No5

Teen Suicide Statistics Sources On-line:

National Institute of Mental Health
http://www.nimh.nih.gov/index.shtml

National Youth Violence
Prevention and Control
http://www.cdc.gov/ViolencePrevention/youthviolence/index.html

National Center for
Injury Prevention and Control
http://www.cdc.gov/injury/

ABOUT THE AUTHOR

Kathy Harris Henderson is a born and bred East Texan. She studied psychology and sociology at Stephen F. Austin State University in Nacogdoches, Texas, then went on to receive a Doctor of Philosophy from Aspen Christian College and Seminary in Dallas.

Following the unexpected and painful loss of her 16 year old daughter, she committed to share what she learned to help both parents and youth understand the importance of forming the type of relationships that ultimately affect behavior and choice. She works to accomplish this in her own church, Greater Mount Pleasant Baptist Church of Dallas, and in the larger community.

Dr. Henderson realizes that so much of what she is today is due to the mentoring she received from her mother, grandmother, great-grandmother and aunt. God is the common thread in all these relationships, the thread she continues to pass on as she seeks the completion of His purpose in her life.

Also from Searchlight Press

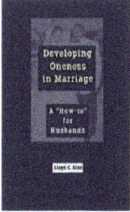

Developing Oneness in Marriage:
A 'How-to' for Husbands
by Rev. Dr. Lloyd C. Blue
(Searchlight Press, 2011)

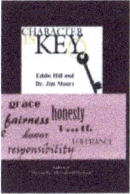

Character Is Key:
In Sports and in Life
by Eddie Hill and Dr. Jim Moore
(Searchlight Press, 2010)

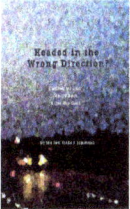

Headed the Wrong Direction?
Calling Us and Others
Back from the Edge
by Rev. Wade J. Simmons
(Searchlight Press, 2011)

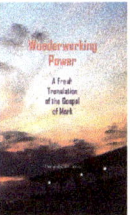

Wonderworking Power:
A Fresh Translation
of the Gospel of Mark
by John Cunyus
(Searchlight Press, 2011)

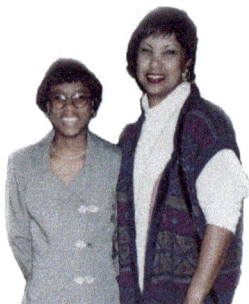

Searchlight Press
Who are you looking for?
Publishers of thoughtful Christian books since 1994.
5634 Ledgestone Drive
Dallas, TX 75214-2026
888.896.6081
info@Searchlight-Press.com
www.Searchlight-Press.com